Radiant Skin;

A Comprehensive Guide to Skincare for Beauty Inside and Out

Table of Contents:

Chapter 1: Introduction to Skincare

1.1 Understanding the Importance of Skincare

Skincare is not just about achieving a flawless complexion or looking good; it plays a crucial role in maintaining the overall health and well-being of our largest organ, which is the skin. Our skin actually serves as a protector from multiple external factors such as pollution, UV radiation, dirt, and pathogens. Proper skincare helps strengthen this barrier, reducing the risk of skin damage and premature aging.

Skincare routines, like cleansing, moisturizing, and exfoliating, are essential for removing dead skin cells, unclogging pores, and promoting healthy cell turnover. This results in a clearer, smoother, and more radiant complexion.

Regular skincare can prevent or manage various skin concerns, such as acne, dryness, redness, and sensitivity. Targeted products and treatments can address specific issues, improving the skin's condition over time.

Proper skincare can slow down the appearance of fine lines, wrinkles, and age spots. Ingredients like retinoids and antioxidants can help stimulate collagen production and protect the skin from free radicals.

Clear, healthy skin can have a positive impact on one's self-esteem and confidence. When you feel good about your skin, you are more likely to feel comfortable and confident in your own skin.

Skincare routines offer an opportunity to take a few moments of self-care amidst our busy lives. Engaging in a soothing skincare ritual can reduce stress and promote a sense of well-being. Using sunscreen regularly is crucial in protecting the skin from harmful UV rays, reducing the risk of skin cancer, and preventing sunburn.

A well-maintained canvas (skin) makes makeup application smoother and enhances the overall look. Skincare can also improve makeup longevity and prevent clogged pores. Investing in preventive skincare can help avoid costly and invasive treatments in the future. Regular maintenance is often more effective and budget-friendly.

In summary, skincare is about nurturing and caring for our skin, not just for its appearance but for its health and function as well. A consistent skincare routine tailored to individual needs can help achieve and maintain healthy, glowing skin throughout life. It is a simple yet powerful way to show ourselves the love and care we deserve.

1.2 The Science Behind Healthy Skin

Our skin is a complex organ that serves as a protective barrier between our internal organs and the outside world. It consists of three primary layers: the epidermis, the dermis, and the subcutaneous tissue. To understand the science behind healthy skin, let's explore the key factors that contribute to its health and function.

Epidermis - The Outermost Layer: The epidermis is the top layer of the skin and acts as a shield against external factors like UV radiation, pollutants, and pathogens. It contains several types of cells, including keratinocytes, which produce the protein keratin that strengthens the skin, and melanocytes, which produce melanin, the pigment that gives our skin its color. The epidermis continuously renews itself through a process called cell turnover. New skin cells are formed at the bottom layer (stratum basale) and gradually move up toward the surface. As old cells shed, new ones take their place, resulting in fresh, healthy-looking skin.

Dermis - The Middle Layer: The dermis is the second layer of the skin and is responsible for providing strength, elasticity, and support. It contains collagen, elastin, and other fibers that give the skin its structure and flexibility. The dermis also houses blood vessels, nerves, hair follicles, and sweat glands.

Collagen and Elastin: Collagen is the most abundant protein in the dermis, providing strength and structural integrity to the skin. Elastin, another protein, allows the skin to snap back into place after being stretched. Both collagen and elastin contribute to the skin's firmness and resilience.

Subcutaneous Tissue - The Innermost Layer: The subcutaneous tissue is the deepest layer of the skin and consists of fat cells that provide insulation and cushioning. This layer plays a role in regulating body temperature and protecting internal organs.

Sebaceous Glands: These glands secrete sebum, an oily substance that lubricates and waterproofs the skin. Sebum helps maintain the skin's natural moisture balance, preventing it from becoming too dry or too oily.

Skin Barrier Function: The outermost layer of the epidermis, known as the stratum corneum, acts as a barrier, preventing water loss and protecting against external irritants. A healthy skin barrier is essential for maintaining hydration and keeping harmful substances out.

Acid Mantle: The skin has a slightly acidic pH, which is referred to as the acid mantle. This acidity helps inhibit the growth of harmful bacteria and fungi, preserving skin health.

Skin Microbiome: The skin is home to a diverse community of microorganisms collectively known as the skin microbiome. This symbiotic relationship helps maintain skin health by contributing to the acid mantle and defending against harmful pathogens.

Inflammatory Response: When the skin is injured or exposed to irritants, the body's inflammatory response is activated. This process helps heal wounds, fight infections, and repair damaged tissues.

To maintain healthy skin, it is essential to protect and support these intricate processes. Proper skincare, a balanced diet, hydration, sun protection, and lifestyle choices all play a significant role in promoting vibrant, healthy skin for a lifetime.

1.3 Debunking Common Skincare Myths

Myth 1: "I don't need sunscreen on cloudy days." Debunked: Clouds do not block UV rays entirely. Even on cloudy days, harmful UVA and UVB rays can still penetrate the clouds and cause skin damage. It's essential to wear sunscreen daily, regardless of the weather.

Myth 2: "Using more skincare products will give better results." Debunked: Overloading your skin with too many products can be counterproductive and may lead to irritation or breakouts. Stick to a simple and effective skincare routine with products tailored to your skin's needs.

Myth 3: "Exfoliating daily is good for my skin." Debunked: Over-exfoliating can strip away the skin's natural protective barrier and lead to sensitivity and irritation. Limit exfoliation to 2-3 times a week, depending on your skin type and the exfoliant's strength.

Myth 4: "Natural ingredients are always better than synthetic ones." Debunked: Natural doesn't always mean better. Many synthetic ingredients are extensively researched and proven to be safe and effective. On the other hand, some natural ingredients can cause allergies or irritation. It's essential to consider the overall formulation and quality of the product.

Myth 5: "Pores can be permanently shrunk or closed." Debunked: Pore size is mainly determined by genetics and can't be permanently changed. However, you can minimize the appearance of pores with proper skincare, like keeping them clean and using products that contain ingredients like salicylic acid.

Myth 6: "You should avoid moisturizer if you have oily skin." Debunked: All skin types need hydration, including oily skin. Skipping moisturizer can actually lead to more oil production as the skin tries to compensate for the lack of moisture. Opt for a lightweight, non-comedogenic moisturizer suited to your skin type.

Myth 7: "You need to use expensive skincare products for results." Debunked: Price doesn't always determine the effectiveness of a product. Many affordable skincare brands offer excellent formulations with scientifically-backed ingredients. Focus on the ingredients and how they suit your skin rather than the price tag.

Myth 8: "Sunscreen is only necessary at the beach or during summer." Debunked: Sunscreen is crucial year-round, regardless of the season or your location. UV rays can still harm your skin even on cool or cloudy days. Always wear sunscreen when you're exposed to daylight.

Myth 9: "You can 'open' or 'close' pores with hot or cold water." Debunked: Pores don't have muscles, so they can't be opened or closed. However, using warm water can help soften sebum and debris, making it easier to cleanse the skin effectively.

Myth 10: "Skincare products can erase wrinkles completely." Debunked: While some skincare products may help reduce the appearance of wrinkles, no topical product can completely erase them. Combining a healthy skincare routine with lifestyle choices can help slow down the aging process.

Remember, understanding the science of skincare and relying on evidence-based information is essential for making informed decisions about your skincare routine.

Chapter 2: Know Your Skin

2.1 Identifying Different Skin Types

There are generally five main skin types, each characterized by specific characteristics and needs. It's essential to identify your skin type accurately to choose the right skincare products and routines for optimal results.

Normal Skin: Normal skin is well-balanced, with an even texture and a good moisture balance. It is neither too oily nor too dry. People with normal skin usually have small pores and few blemishes. Their complexion is generally clear and smooth.

Dry Skin: Dry skin lacks moisture and often feels tight and flaky. It may appear dull and rough, with visible fine lines and a tendency to develop dry patches. People with dry skin may experience discomfort and irritation, especially in harsh weather conditions.

Oily Skin: Oily skin produces an excess of sebum, resulting in a shiny appearance, particularly in the T-zone (forehead, nose, and chin). Individuals with oily skin often have larger pores and are more prone to acne and breakouts.

Combination Skin: Combination skin is a mix of different skin types. Typically, the T-zone is oilier, while the cheeks and other areas may be normal to dry. Managing combination skin may require using different products for different areas of the face.

Sensitive Skin: Sensitive skin is easily irritated and reacts to various skincare products or environmental factors. It may experience redness, itching, and a burning sensation. People with sensitive skin need gentle, fragrance-free products to avoid irritation.

It's important to note that skin types can change over time due to factors such as age, hormonal changes, climate, and lifestyle. Therefore, regularly reassessing your skin type and adjusting your skincare routine accordingly is crucial for maintaining healthy, balanced skin.

2.2 Common Skin Concerns and Solutions

Acne

Use a gentle cleanser twice daily, avoid touching your face, and refrain from picking or squeezing pimples. Incorporate products with ingredients like salicylic acid or benzoyl peroxide to target acne-causing bacteria. Consult a dermatologist for severe cases.

Dryness

Hydrate your skin with a moisturizer suitable for your skin type. Avoid hot showers and use a humidifier in dry environments. Choose products containing hyaluronic acid and glycerin to lock in moisture.

Hyperpigmentation (Dark Spots)

Apply sunscreen daily to prevent further darkening. Use products with ingredients like vitamin C, niacinamide, or retinoids to fade dark spots over time. Consider chemical peels or laser treatments for more severe cases.

Fine Lines and Wrinkles

Incorporate anti-aging products with retinol or peptides into your skincare routine. Use sunscreen daily to protect against photoaging. Consider procedures like microdermabrasion or microneedling for advanced anti-aging benefits.

Oily Skin and Enlarged Pores

Use oil-free or mattifying products to control excess oil. Consider toners containing witch hazel or salicylic acid to minimize pore appearance. Regularly exfoliate to prevent clogged pores.

Redness and Sensitivity

Choose gentle, fragrance-free products suitable for sensitive skin. Incorporate products with soothing ingredients like

aloe vera, chamomile, or green tea extract. Avoid hot water and
harsh exfoliants.

Uneven Skin Tone

Use brightening agents like vitamin C or kojic acid to even
out skin tone. Exfoliate regularly to promote cell turnover. Apply
sunscreen to prevent further hyperpigmentation.

Under Eye Circles and Puffiness

Get enough sleep and stay hydrated. Use an eye cream with
ingredients like caffeine or hyaluronic acid to reduce puffiness.
Consider cool compresses to soothe tired eyes.

Dull Skin

Exfoliate regularly to remove dead skin cells and promote
skin radiance. Use products with ingredients like alpha hydroxy
acids (AHAs) or vitamin C to boost skin brightness. Stay hydrated
and get enough sleep.

Blackheads

Use a gentle exfoliant with salicylic acid to unclog pores.
Consider using a clay mask once a week to absorb excess oil. Avoid
squeezing or picking at blackheads to prevent irritation and
scarring.

Remember that skincare solutions may vary depending on
individual skin types and conditions. It's essential to establish a
consistent and personalized skincare routine and seek advice from a
dermatologist for persistent or severe skin concerns.

Chapter 3: The Essential Skincare Routine

3.1 Cleansing: The Foundation of Beautiful Skin

Cleansing your skin properly is a fundamental step in any skincare routine. It helps remove dirt, makeup, excess oil, and impurities, ensuring that your skin is clean and ready to successfully absorb further skincare products. Start by washing your hands thoroughly with soap and water. This step ensures that you're not transferring any dirt or bacteria to your face during the cleansing process. If you're wearing makeup, use a makeup remover or a gentle cleansing oil to dissolve and remove it from your skin. You can also use micellar water or makeup wipes for this purpose. Use warm water to loosen and dissolve any oil inside the pores. Select a cleanser suitable for your skin type. If you have dry or sensitive skin, go for a gentle, hydrating cleanser. For oily or acne-prone skin, opt for a foaming or gel-based cleanser that helps control excess oil. Splash your face with lukewarm water to prepare it for cleansing. Avoid using hot water, as it can strip the skin of its natural oils and cause dryness. Take a small amount of the cleanser and gently massage it onto your damp face in circular motions. Focus on areas prone to oiliness or makeup buildup, such as the forehead, nose, and chin. Be gentle; Avoid scrubbing your face vigorously, especially if you have sensitive skin. Be gentle and use light pressure to avoid irritation. After cleansing, rinse your face thoroughly with lukewarm water. Make sure there's no residue left on your skin. Pat Dry; Gently pat your face dry with a soft, clean towel. Avoid rubbing your skin, as it can lead to irritation and excessive redness. If you use a toner as part of your skincare routine, apply it after cleansing. Toners can help balance the skin's pH and prepare it for the next steps. After cleansing and toning (if applicable), continue with the rest of your skincare routine, such as serums, moisturizers, and sunscreen.

Cleanse your skin twice a day, in the morning and evening, to maintain a clean and healthy complexion. If you have dry or sensitive skin, you may choose to cleanse once a day in the evening.

Remember to choose products suitable for your skin type and avoid harsh ingredients that may cause irritation. Consistent and proper cleansing is key to keeping your skin clean, clear, and ready to absorb the benefits of your skincare products.

3.2 Exfoliation: Revealing Fresh Radiance

Exfoliating your face is an essential step in your skincare routine that helps remove dead skin cells, unclog pores, and promote a brighter and smoother complexion. Here's a step-by-step guide on how to exfoliate your face effectively:

Choose the Right Exfoliant: There are two main types of exfoliants: physical exfoliants with scrubbing particles and chemical exfoliants with active ingredients like alpha hydroxy acids (AHAs) or beta hydroxy acids (BHAs). Choose the one that suits your skin type and concerns.

Physical and chemical facial exfoliants are both skincare products designed to remove dead skin cells and promote a smoother, brighter complexion, but they achieve this through different mechanisms. Here's a breakdown of the differences between the two:

Physical Exfoliants: Also known as mechanical exfoliants, physical exfoliants contain small particles or granules that physically scrub away dead skin cells when massaged onto the skin. These particles can be natural materials like sugar, salt, rice bran, or ground fruit pits, or they can be synthetic materials like microbeads. The exfoliation occurs due to the abrasive action of these particles rubbing against the skin's surface.

Pros of Physical Exfoliants:

1. Immediate texture improvement: Physical exfoliants can provide an instant feeling of smoother skin.

2. Physical sensation: Some people enjoy the tactile experience of using scrubs and feeling the exfoliation process.

3. Visible results: The removal of dead skin cells can lead to a temporary improvement in skin texture and appearance.

Cons of Physical Exfoliants:

1. Harshness: Some physical exfoliants can be too abrasive, leading to micro-tears in the skin or irritation, especially if used too vigorously or on sensitive skin.

2. Uneven exfoliation: It's easy to apply uneven pressure or miss certain areas, leading to inconsistent results.

3. Potential for overuse: Regular use of harsh physical exfoliants can disrupt the skin's barrier function and lead to irritation, redness, and dryness.

Chemical Exfoliants: Chemical exfoliants utilize acids or enzymes to dissolve the bonds between dead skin cells, encouraging their removal. There are two main types of chemical exfoliants:

1. **Alpha Hydroxy Acids (AHAs):** These include glycolic acid (from sugarcane), lactic acid (from milk), and mandelic acid (from almonds). They work on the skin's surface, helping to exfoliate dead cells and improve skin texture.

2. **Beta Hydroxy Acids (BHAs):** Salicylic acid is a common BHA. It penetrates deeper into the pores, making it effective for those with oily or acne-prone skin. BHAs can help exfoliate the interior of pores and reduce the appearance of blackheads and breakouts.

Pros of Chemical Exfoliants:

1. Controlled exfoliation: Chemical exfoliants can provide more consistent and controlled exfoliation without the risk of over-scrubbing.

2. Deeper penetration: Chemical exfoliants can reach areas that physical exfoliants might miss, like inside pores.

3. Mildness: When used correctly, chemical exfoliants can be gentler on the skin's surface than some harsh physical exfoliants.

Cons of Chemical Exfoliants:

1. Sensitivity: Some people with sensitive skin might experience irritation or redness when using chemical exfoliants, especially if they're not introduced gradually.

2. Photosensitivity: Chemical exfoliants can increase the skin's sensitivity to sunlight, so proper sun protection is crucial when using them.

3. Gradual results: While chemical exfoliants can provide long-term benefits, they might not give the immediate sensation of smoothness that physical exfoliants do.

In summary, the choice between physical and chemical exfoliants depends on your skin type, concerns, and preferences. It's important to choose products that are appropriate for your skin's needs and to use them in moderation to avoid over-exfoliation and potential skin damage. If you're uncertain, consulting a dermatologist can help you determine the best exfoliation approach for your skin.

Before exfoliating, cleanse your face with a gentle cleanser to remove any makeup, dirt, or excess oil. Pat your skin dry with a clean towel. How often you should exfoliate depends on your skin type. For most skin types, exfoliating 2-3 times a week is sufficient. If you have sensitive skin, consider exfoliating less frequently (once a week) or using a milder exfoliant.

Physical Exfoliation:

1. Take a small amount of the physical exfoliant on your fingertips.

2. Gently massage the exfoliant onto your damp face using circular motions. Avoid the eye area and be gentle with your movements.

3. Focus on areas prone to roughness or congestion, such as the forehead, nose, and chin.

4. Rinse your face thoroughly with lukewarm water to remove the exfoliant completely.

Chemical Exfoliation:

1. Apply a small amount of the chemical exfoliant to a clean, dry face. Start with a lower concentration if you're new to chemical exfoliants.
2. Avoid the eye area and be careful not to over-apply the product.
3. Let the chemical exfoliant sit on your skin for the recommended time (usually a few minutes) according to the product's instructions.
4. Rinse your face with lukewarm water to neutralize the exfoliant, or follow the product's instructions on leaving it on the skin.
5. Moisturize: After exfoliating, it's crucial to apply a hydrating moisturizer to replenish the skin's moisture barrier.

Exfoliating can make your skin more sensitive to the sun. Always apply sunscreen with at least SPF 30 during the day to protect your skin from harmful UV rays. Pay attention to how your skin responds to exfoliation. If you experience redness, irritation, or excessive dryness, reduce the frequency of exfoliation or try a milder exfoliant.

Remember, exfoliating too frequently or using harsh products can damage the skin's protective barrier and lead to sensitivity. Be gentle and consistent with your exfoliation routine to achieve a healthy and radiant complexion. If you're unsure which exfoliant is right for you, consult with a dermatologist or skincare professional.

3.3 Toning: Balancing and Preparing the Skin

A toner is a liquid skincare product designed to be applied to the face after cleansing and before moisturizing. Toners offer various benefits and play an essential role in a well-rounded skincare routine. Here's what a toner does for your face:

Balances pH Levels: Cleansers, especially foaming ones, can disrupt the skin's natural pH balance. Toners help restore the skin's pH, creating an environment where the skin can function optimally.

Cleansing Residue Removal: Toners can help remove any leftover traces of dirt, makeup, or cleanser that might have been missed during the cleansing process. This ensures the skin is clean and ready to absorb subsequent skincare products.

Tightens and Shrinks Pores: Some toners contain astringent properties that temporarily tighten and minimize the appearance of pores. This can give the skin a smoother and more refined look.

Hydration and Moisture: Many toners are formulated with hydrating ingredients like hyaluronic acid or glycerin. They help attract and retain moisture, keeping the skin hydrated and plump.

Soothing and Calming: Toners with ingredients like chamomile, aloe vera, or green tea extract can have soothing properties that calm red or irritated skin.

Enhances Absorption: Applying toner before other skincare products can enhance their absorption. It creates a slightly damp surface for serums and moisturizers to penetrate more effectively.

Preparation for Active Ingredients: If you use serums or treatments with active ingredients like retinoids or AHAs, toners can help prepare the skin for better absorption, minimizing potential irritation.

Refreshes the Skin: Applying a toner can provide a refreshing and invigorating sensation, especially when the toner contains natural extracts like citrus or mint.

Antioxidant Protection: Some toners contain antioxidants like vitamin C or green tea, which help protect the skin from free radical damage caused by environmental stressors.

Customization: Toners are available for various skin types and concerns, allowing you to choose one that suits your specific needs, such as toners for oily skin, sensitive skin, or acne-prone skin.

To use a toner, simply pour a small amount onto a cotton pad or into your hands and gently pat or sweep it across your face and neck. Allow the toner to dry before proceeding with the rest of your skincare routine. Remember that toners are not a necessary step for everyone, but they can be beneficial for many skin types, especially when tailored to specific needs.

3.4 Moisturizing: Nourishing the Skin Barrier

Moisturizing and nourishing your face are essential steps in a skincare routine to keep your skin hydrated, healthy, and radiant. Here's what you need to know about moisturizing and nourishing your face:

Choose the right moisturizer. Select a moisturizer that suits your skin type and addresses your specific concerns. For dry skin, opt for a rich, hydrating moisturizer, while those with oily skin should look for lightweight, oil-free options. Consistency is key; Moisturizing and nourishing your face should be part of your daily skincare routine. Consistency is crucial to maintaining healthy and radiant skin.

Always apply on damp skin. After cleansing and toning, apply your moisturizer while your skin is still slightly damp. This helps lock in moisture and ensures better absorption. If your moisturizer doesn't contain SPF, layer it with a broad-spectrum sunscreen of at least SPF 30 during the day to protect your skin from UV rays. Consider using a separate night cream, which is often richer and formulated to provide extra hydration and nourishment while you sleep. Look for moisturizers containing hyaluronic acid, a powerful humectant that attracts and retains moisture in the skin. Antioxidants like vitamin C, vitamin E, or green tea extract are also beneficial in your routine. Antioxidants protect the skin from free radicals, which can cause premature aging. Nourish your skin with products containing essential fatty acids like omega-3 and omega-6. These help strengthen the skin's barrier and maintain moisture balance.Skincare products with vitamins and minerals also promote skin health, such as vitamin A (retinol), vitamin B3 (niacinamide), and zinc. Consider using facial oils to provide an extra boost of nourishment. Oils like rosehip oil, jojoba oil, or argan oil can be beneficial for different skin types. You also can periodically use sheet masks enriched with serums containing beneficial ingredients like aloe vera, collagen, or hyaluronic acid for a quick and intense nourishing treatment.

Remember, everyone's skin is unique, so it's essential to find products that work well for your specific skin type and concerns. If you have specific skin conditions or concerns, consider consulting with a dermatologist or skincare professional for personalized advice and recommendations.

3.5 Sunscreen: Shielding from Harmful UV Rays

Sunscreen is of utmost importance for your face and should be an essential part of your daily skincare routine. Here are some key reasons why sunscreen is crucial for protecting and maintaining the health of your facial skin:

1. Protection from Harmful UV Rays: Sunscreen acts as a shield, protecting your skin from the damaging effects of ultraviolet (UV) rays from the sun. UV rays can cause various skin issues, including sunburn, premature aging (wrinkles, fine lines, and age spots), and an increased risk of skin cancer.

2. Prevents Sunburn: Sunscreen helps prevent sunburn, which is not only painful and uncomfortable but also a sign of skin damage from excessive UV exposure.

3. Reduces the Risk of Skin Cancer: Prolonged and unprotected exposure to UV rays is a significant risk factor for skin cancer, including melanoma, the deadliest form of skin cancer. Regularly applying sunscreen can significantly lower this risk.

4. Prevents Premature Aging: UV rays can break down collagen and elastin in the skin, leading to premature aging and the formation of wrinkles and sagging skin. Sunscreen helps maintain the skin's firmness and youthful appearance.

5. Prevents Hyperpigmentation: Sunscreen can help prevent the overproduction of melanin, which leads to hyperpigmentation (dark spots) on the skin.

6. Protection from Photoaging: Photoaging is skin aging caused by UV exposure. Sunscreen acts as a powerful anti-aging tool, preventing photoaging and maintaining a more youthful complexion.

7. Maintains Even Skin Tone: Sunscreen helps prevent uneven skin tone and discoloration caused by sun damage, keeping your complexion more even and radiant.

8. Combats Skin Sensitivity: Sunscreen can help protect and soothe sensitive skin, reducing redness and irritation caused by sun exposure.

9. Preserves Skincare Results: If you're using products with active ingredients like retinoids or vitamin C, sunscreen is vital to protect and preserve their effectiveness.

UV rays are present all year, even on cloudy days and during winter. Therefore, wearing sunscreen daily, regardless of the weather, is essential for continuous protection. To get the full benefits of sunscreen, choose a broad-spectrum sunscreen with SPF 30 or higher. Apply it generously to your face and exposed areas at least 15-30 minutes before sun exposure. Reapply every two hours, especially if you're sweating or swimming. Remember, sun protection is a crucial aspect of maintaining healthy, youthful, and beautiful skin.

Chapter 4: The Power of Skincare Ingredients

4.1 Antioxidants: Combatting Free Radicals

Combatting free radicals is essential for maintaining healthy and youthful skin. Free radicals are unstable molecules that can damage skin cells and accelerate the aging process.

Antioxidants help neutralize free radicals, preventing them from causing harm to your skin. Look for skincare products containing antioxidants such as vitamin C, vitamin E, green tea extract, niacinamide, resveratrol, or coenzyme Q10.Remember, sunscreen is your first line of defense against free radical damage caused by UV radiation. Apply a broad-spectrum sunscreen with at least SPF 30 daily, even on cloudy days, to protect your skin from harmful UV rays. Limit your time in the sun, especially during peak hours (10 a.m. to 4 p.m.). Seeking shade and wearing protective clothing, hats, and sunglasses can further reduce exposure. Quit smoking; Smoking is a significant source of free radicals. Quitting smoking not only benefits your overall health but also helps protect your skin from premature aging caused by smoking-related free radicals. Consume a diet rich in antioxidants from fruits, vegetables, nuts, and seeds. Foods high in vitamins A, C, and E, as well as selenium and zinc, support the skin's natural defense against free radicals.

Drinking enough water helps flush out toxins from your body, aiding in the fight against free radicals.Limit alcohol and caffeine. Excessive alcohol and caffeine consumption can increase free radical production. Moderation is key to minimizing their impact on your skin.

Manage Stress: Chronic stress can contribute to free radical formation. Practice stress-reducing techniques such as meditation, yoga, or spending time in nature.

Sleep Well: Proper sleep allows your body to repair and regenerate, reducing the accumulation of free radical damage.

Gentle Skincare: Avoid harsh skincare products that may irritate your skin and lead to increased free radical production. Stick to gentle, non-irritating formulations.

A combination of internal and external approaches is necessary to combat free radicals effectively. By incorporating antioxidants, sun protection, a healthy lifestyle, and a well-balanced skincare routine, you can help keep your skin looking youthful and radiant while protecting it from environmental stressors.

4.2 Hyaluronic Acid: The Ultimate Hydrator

Hyaluronic acid is a popular skincare ingredient known for its excellent hydrating properties. When used correctly, it can significantly benefit your skin. Hyaluronic acid is a humectant, which means it attracts and retains water. It can hold up to 1000 times its weight in water, making it incredibly effective at hydrating the skin. When your skin is well-hydrated, it appears plumper and smoother, reducing the appearance of fine lines and wrinkles. Hyaluronic acid is generally well-tolerated and suitable for all skin types, including sensitive and acne-prone skin. Hyaluronic acid has a lightweight and non-greasy texture, making it easy to incorporate into your skincare routine. By providing essential hydration, hyaluronic acid helps strengthen the skin's barrier, protecting it from external irritants and pollutants. Dehydrated skin can look dull and lackluster. Hyaluronic acid helps revive and rejuvenate the skin, giving it a healthy, radiant appearance, and can be easily incorporated into your existing skincare routine. It works well with other active ingredients like vitamin C, retinol, and peptides.

Remember to patch-test new products containing hyaluronic acid before applying them to your entire face, especially if you have sensitive skin or are trying a new brand. As with any skincare product, consistency is key. Incorporate hyaluronic acid into your daily routine to experience its long-term hydrating benefits.

4.3 Retinoids: The Miracle Anti-Ager

Retinoids are a class of chemical compounds derived from vitamin A. They are used in skincare for their numerous benefits and are considered one of the most effective ingredients for addressing various skin concerns. Retinoids work by promoting skin cell turnover and collagen production. Here's what you need to know about retinoids:

Types of Retinoids: There are various types of retinoids used in skincare, ranging from mild to potent. Some common retinoids include retinol, retinaldehyde, tretinoin (retinoic acid), adapalene, and tazarotene. Retinoids are known for their anti-aging properties. They help reduce the appearance of fine lines, wrinkles, and age spots by stimulating collagen production and increasing skin cell turnover. Retinoids are even effective in treating acne by unclogging pores, reducing inflammation, and preventing the formation of new acne lesions. Regular use of retinoids can lead to smoother, more even skin texture and a more radiant complexion, and can help fade dark spots and hyperpigmentation by promoting skin cell turnover and reducing melanin production. Retinoids help to exfoliate the skin, which can unclog pores and reduce the formation of blackheads and whiteheads.

Prescription vs. Over-the-Counter (OTC) Retinoids: Some retinoids, such as tretinoin and tazarotene, are available by prescription and are more potent. Over-the-counter retinoids, like retinol and retinaldehyde, are generally milder and can be suitable for those new to using retinoids.

When using retinoids for the first time, it's essential to start slowly and gradually increase usage. They can cause some initial irritation, redness, and peeling, but this often subsides as your skin adjusts. Retinoids are best used at night because they can make the skin more sensitive to sunlight. Applying them before bedtime allows your skin to reap the benefits while you sleep.

When using retinoids, it's essential to avoid using products with exfoliating ingredients like alpha hydroxy acids (AHAs) and beta hydroxy acids (BHAs) on the same days to prevent over-exfoliation and irritation.

Retinoids can be highly effective in addressing various skin concerns, but they are not suitable for everyone. If you have sensitive skin or certain medical conditions, it's best to consult with a dermatologist before incorporating retinoids into your skincare routine.

4.4 Vitamin C: The Brightening Agent

Vitamin C is a powerful antioxidant that offers numerous benefits for your face and skin. It is a popular skincare ingredient known for its ability to brighten, protect, and promote a more youthful complexion. Here's why vitamin C is beneficial for your face:

1. Antioxidant Protection: Vitamin C is a potent antioxidant that helps neutralize free radicals, which are unstable molecules that can damage skin cells and contribute to premature aging.

2. Brightens the Skin: Vitamin C has skin-brightening properties, helping to even out skin tone and reduce the appearance of dark spots and hyperpigmentation.

3. Boosts Collagen Production: Vitamin C is essential for collagen synthesis, a protein that gives the skin its firmness and elasticity. By promoting collagen production, vitamin C can help minimize the appearance of fine lines and wrinkles.

4. Reduces Inflammation: Vitamin C has anti-inflammatory properties that can soothe redness and irritation, making it beneficial for sensitive or acne-prone skin.

5. Enhances Sun Protection: While vitamin C is not a replacement for sunscreen, it can complement sun protection efforts by neutralizing free radicals caused by UV exposure.

6. Improves Skin Texture: Regular use of vitamin C can lead to smoother and more supple skin, thanks to its role in collagen synthesis and exfoliation.

7. Supports Wound Healing: Vitamin C aids in the skin's natural healing process, making it beneficial for post-inflammatory hyperpigmentation and helping wounds and blemishes heal faster.

8. Suitable for Most Skin Types: Vitamin C is generally well-tolerated by most skin types, including sensitive skin. However, some people may experience slight irritation or sensitivity, especially when using high concentrations of vitamin C.

To incorporate vitamin C into your skincare routine, you can use products like serums, moisturizers, or creams containing vitamin C. Look for stable forms of vitamin C, such as L-ascorbic acid, as this form tends to be more effective. Start with a lower concentration and gradually increase as your skin builds tolerance. Vitamin C is most effective when applied in the morning before sunscreen, as it enhances protection against environmental damage throughout the day. As with any new skincare product, it's a good idea to patch-test vitamin C products before applying them to your entire face, especially if you have sensitive skin. If you're unsure about which vitamin C product to use or have specific skin concerns, consider consulting with a dermatologist for personalized recommendations.

4.5 Natural Extracts and Botanicals

There are numerous natural extracts and botanicals that are commonly used in skincare products due to their potential beneficial properties. Here are some examples:

1. **Aloe Vera:** Known for its soothing and hydrating properties, aloe vera can help calm irritated skin and provide moisture.

2. **Chamomile:** Chamomile has anti-inflammatory and antioxidant properties, making it useful for soothing sensitive or irritated skin.

3. **Green Tea:** Rich in antioxidants, green tea can help protect the skin from environmental damage and reduce inflammation.

4. **Rosehip Oil:** Derived from the seeds of wild rose bushes, rosehip oil is high in vitamins and essential fatty acids that promote skin regeneration and hydration.

5. **Lavender:** Lavender oil is often used for its calming scent, and it also has potential antibacterial and anti-inflammatory effects.

6. **Calendula:** Calendula extract is known for its soothing and anti-inflammatory properties, making it suitable for sensitive or dry skin.

7. **Witch Hazel:** Witch hazel is an astringent with potential benefits for toning the skin, reducing inflammation, and tightening pores.

8. **Jojoba Oil:** Jojoba oil closely resembles the skin's natural sebum and can help balance oil production while providing hydration.

9. **Hyaluronic Acid:** While not a botanical, hyaluronic acid is a naturally occurring substance in the body that helps retain moisture, making it a popular choice for hydrating skincare products.

10. **Coconut Oil:** Coconut oil is often used for its moisturizing properties, but it's important to note that it can be comedogenic (pore-clogging) for some individuals.

11. **Oat Extract:** Oat extract is known for its soothing and anti-itch properties, making it useful for calming irritated or inflamed skin.

12. **Ginseng:** Ginseng has potential anti-aging properties and can help improve the appearance of skin tone and texture.

13. **Turmeric:** Turmeric contains curcumin, which has anti-inflammatory and antioxidant properties. It's used to brighten the complexion and soothe skin.

14. **Sea Buckthorn Oil:** This oil is rich in vitamins, minerals, and fatty acids, making it beneficial for promoting skin hydration and elasticity.

15. **Cucumber Extract:** Cucumber has a cooling and hydrating effect on the skin, making it useful for soothing puffiness and irritation.

16. **Licorice Root Extract:** Licorice root can help reduce redness and hyperpigmentation, making it suitable for those with uneven skin tone.

17. **Moringa Oil:** Moringa oil is rich in antioxidants and nutrients that can help nourish and protect the skin from environmental stressors. ype, concerns, and preferences. It's important to choose products that are appropriate for your skin's needs and to use them in moderation to avoid over-exfoliation and potential skin damage. If you're uncertain, consulting a dermatologist can help you determine the best exfoliation approach for your skin.

When incorporating natural extracts and botanicals into your skincare routine, it's important to patch-test new products to ensure you don't have any adverse reactions, especially if you have sensitive skin or allergies. Additionally, it's a good idea to consult with a dermatologist or skincare professional, especially if you have specific skin concerns or conditions.

Chapter 5: Customizing Your Skincare Routine

5.1 Adapting Skincare for Different Seasons

Adapting your skincare routine for different seasons is essential because environmental factors can have varying effects on your skin throughout the year. Here are some tips to adjust your skincare routine for each season.

In the springtime, transition to lighter formulas: As the weather warms up, switch to lighter moisturizers and serums that won't feel heavy on the skin. Include products with antioxidants like vitamin C to protect your skin from increased sun exposure and environmental pollutants. After the drier winter months, incorporate gentle exfoliation to remove dead skin cells and reveal a fresh complexion.

In the summertime, increase sunscreen protection, as the sun's UV rays are stronger, so use a broad-spectrum sunscreen with a higher SPF to shield your skin from damage. Despite the heat, your skin may still need hydration. Opt for lightweight, oil-free moisturizers to prevent clogged pores. If you have oily skin, use oil-absorbing products like mattifying primers or blotting papers to manage excess shine.

In the fall, start with repairing any sun damage from the summer with products containing ingredients like niacinamide or hyaluronic acid. Consider incorporating retinoids into your routine during fall, as the weather becomes cooler and less humid. Start with a lower concentration to avoid excessive dryness. As the air gets drier, prioritize hydrating products and consider using a humidifier indoors to maintain moisture.

Winter air is often dry, which can lead to skin dehydration. Use richer moisturizers and oils to lock in moisture. Don't forget to keep your lips hydrated with lip balms or treatments. You may want to shield your face from harsh winter elements by wearing scarves or using a face mask.

5.2 Tailoring Skincare for Age Groups

Skincare needs can vary depending on your age group, as different life stages come with specific skin concerns and priorities. Here's a general overview of skincare tips for each age group:

Teenagers (Ages 13-19):

Focus on Cleansing: Teenagers often experience increased oil production and acne. Use a gentle cleanser twice daily to keep the skin clean without stripping it of essential moisture.

Avoid Harsh Products: Steer clear of harsh or abrasive products, as they can irritate the skin and exacerbate acne.

Sunscreen: Start using a broad-spectrum sunscreen daily to protect the skin from UV damage and prevent premature aging.

20-29:

Consistent Routine: Establish a consistent skincare routine with a gentle cleanser, moisturizer, and sunscreen.

Antioxidants: Consider adding products with antioxidants like vitamin C to protect the skin from environmental damage.

Preventive Care: Start using retinoids or retinol to address early signs of aging and promote skin cell turnover.

30-39

Hydration: Focus on hydrating the skin with moisturizers containing hyaluronic acid and ceramides.

Eye Cream: Consider incorporating an eye cream to address fine lines and prevent the appearance of crow's feet.

Sun Protection: Continue using sunscreen daily to prevent sun-induced aging.

40-49:

Targeted Treatments: Add targeted treatments such as peptides and growth factors to address specific concerns like loss of firmness and elasticity.

Exfoliation: Consider gentle exfoliation to promote skin cell turnover and improve skin texture.

Neck and Décolletage Care: Extend your skincare routine to include the neck and décolletage to prevent signs of aging in these areas.

5. 50s and Beyond:

Rich Moisturizers: Use richer, nourishing moisturizers to combat dryness and maintain skin suppleness.

Regular Exfoliation: Continue gentle exfoliation to promote cell turnover and improve skin radiance.

Hydration: Consider adding a hydrating serum or facial oil to your routine for an extra boost of moisture.

Collagen-Boosting Ingredients: Look for products with ingredients like peptides and growth factors to support collagen production and firm the skin.

Remember that individual skin concerns can vary within each age group, and these guidelines are meant to provide a general overview. Tailor your skincare routine based on your specific skin type, concerns, and goals. If you're unsure about what products to use, consider consulting with a dermatologist or skincare professional for personalized recommendations.

5.3 Targeting Specific Skin Concerns

Targeting specific skin concerns requires a personalized approach based on your individual skin type and issues. Here are some common skin concerns and tips on how to address them:

1. Acne-Prone Skin:

-Use a gentle cleanser to keep the skin clean without causing irritation.

-Incorporate products with salicylic acid or benzoyl peroxide to help control acne and reduce inflammation.

-Avoid heavy, pore-clogging moisturizers and opt for oil-free or non-comedogenic options.

-Consider using a retinoid to prevent clogged pores and promote skin cell turnover.

2. Dry Skin:

-Choose a hydrating cleanser that doesn't strip the skin of its natural oils.

-Use a rich, emollient moisturizer to lock in moisture and soothe dryness.

-Look for products containing hyaluronic acid, glycerin, and ceramides to hydrate and strengthen the skin's barrier.

-Consider using a facial oil to provide an extra layer of nourishment and hydration.

3. Oily Skin:

-Use a gentle, oil-free cleanser to remove excess oil without over-drying the skin.

-Look for lightweight, oil-free moisturizers or gel-based formulas to hydrate the skin without adding extra shine.

-Consider using products with niacinamide or witch hazel to help control excess oil production.

4. Dark Spots and Hyperpigmentation:

-Use a broad-spectrum sunscreen daily to prevent further darkening of hyperpigmented areas.

-Incorporate products with ingredients like vitamin C, kojic acid, or alpha arbutin to brighten and fade dark spots.

-Consider using chemical exfoliants with glycolic acid or lactic acid to promote cell turnover and reduce pigmentation.

5. Fine Lines and Wrinkles:

-Use products with retinoids or retinol to stimulate collagen production and reduce the appearance of fine lines and wrinkles.

-Incorporate antioxidants like vitamin C and E to protect the skin from free radical damage.

-Hydrate the skin with moisturizers containing hyaluronic acid to plump and smooth the skin.

6. Dull and Uneven Skin Tone:

-Exfoliate regularly to remove dead skin cells and reveal a brighter complexion.

-Use products with vitamin C or alpha hydroxy acids (AHAs) to promote skin radiance and even out skin tone.

-Consider incorporating a brightening mask or serum for an extra boost of radiance.

7. Sensitive Skin:

-Look for fragrance-free and hypoallergenic products to minimize potential irritation.

-Use gentle, soothing ingredients like aloe vera, chamomile, or oat extract to calm sensitive skin.

-Patch-test new products before applying them to your entire face to check for any adverse reactions.

-Remember that consistent and patient use of targeted products is essential to see improvements in your skin concerns. It's also a good idea to introduce new products one at a time to ensure that your skin doesn't react negatively. If you're unsure about which products to use or how to address specific concerns, consult with a dermatologist or skincare professional for personalized advice and recommendations.

5.4 DIY Skincare at Home

DIY skincare at home can be a fun and cost-effective way to pamper your skin with natural ingredients. However, it's essential to use safe and suitable ingredients for your skin type. Here are some DIY skincare recipes and tips:

1. Honey and Yogurt Face Mask (Hydrating and Soothing):

Mix 1 tablespoon of raw honey with 1 tablespoon of plain yogurt.

Apply the mixture to your face and leave it on for 15-20 minutes.

Rinse off with warm water, and enjoy hydrated and soothed skin.

2. Oatmeal and Milk Cleanser (Gentle Cleansing):

Blend 1 tablespoon of ground oatmeal with 2 tablespoons of milk to create a paste.

Massage the mixture onto your face in circular motions.

Rinse off with water, leaving your skin clean and nourished.

3. Cucumber and Aloe Vera Toner (Refreshing and Calming):

Blend half a cucumber and strain the juice.

Mix the cucumber juice with 2 tablespoons of pure aloe vera gel.

Apply the toner to your face using a cotton ball and let it dry naturally.

4. Coffee Grounds and Coconut Oil Scrub (Exfoliating):

Combine 1 tablespoon of coffee grounds with 1 tablespoon of melted coconut oil.

Gently massage the scrub onto damp skin in circular motions, focusing on areas with rough texture.

Rinse thoroughly and enjoy smoother skin.

5. Green Tea and Lemon Facial Mist (Refreshing and Brightening):

Brew a cup of green tea and let it cool.

Add a few drops of lemon juice to the green tea and transfer it to a spray bottle.

Spritz the mist on your face throughout the day for a refreshing pick-me-up.

Tips for DIY Skincare:

Always do a patch test before applying any DIY skincare product to your entire face to check for allergies or adverse reactions.

Use high-quality, natural ingredients, and avoid anything that may irritate your skin.

If you have sensitive or acne-prone skin, be cautious with certain ingredients that may exacerbate these conditions, like lemon juice or essential oils.

Hygiene is crucial; make sure your hands and tools are clean before starting any DIY skincare process.

Keep in mind that DIY skincare may not offer the same efficacy as commercially formulated products, especially for treating specific skin concerns.

While DIY skincare can be enjoyable and provide some benefits, it's essential to supplement it with a well-balanced skincare routine that includes professionally formulated products for more targeted results. If you have specific skin concerns, it's a good idea to consult with a dermatologist or skincare professional for personalized advice and recommendations.

Chapter 6: The Mind-Skin Connection

6.1 Stress and Its Impact on the Skin

Stress can have a significant impact on the skin, just as it does on your health, leading to various skin issues and exacerbating existing skin conditions. The mind and skin are closely connected through the body's stress response, hormonal changes, and immune system. Here are some ways in which stress can affect the skin:

Acne and Breakouts: Stress triggers the release of stress hormones like cortisol, which can stimulate the oil glands in the skin, leading to increased sebum (oil) production. Excess oil can clog pores and contribute to acne breakouts.

Worsening of Skin Conditions: Stress can worsen existing skin conditions, such as eczema, psoriasis, and rosacea. It can cause flare-ups, redness, and itching in these conditions.

Premature Aging: Chronic stress can accelerate the aging process by promoting inflammation and free radical damage. This can lead to the formation of wrinkles, fine lines, and a dull complexion.

Dryness and Dehydration: Stress can disrupt the skin's barrier function, leading to increased water loss and dry, dehydrated skin.

Dark Circles and Puffy Eyes: Lack of sleep and increased stress can lead to the appearance of dark circles and puffiness around the eyes.

Impaired Skin Healing: Stress can slow down the skin's ability to heal from wounds, cuts, or blemishes.

Skin Sensitivity: Stress can make the skin more reactive and sensitive to external irritants and allergens.

Nail and Hair Issues: Stress can lead to brittle nails, hair loss, or changes in hair texture.

Tips to Manage Stress and Improve Skin Health:

Practice Stress-Relief Techniques: Engage in activities that help you relax and reduce stress, such as meditation, yoga, deep breathing exercises, or spending time in nature.

Prioritize Sleep: Aim for 7-9 hours of quality sleep each night to allow the skin to repair and regenerate.

Regular Exercise: Physical activity can help reduce stress and improve circulation, benefiting the skin.

Healthy Diet: Eat a balanced diet rich in fruits, vegetables, whole grains, and lean proteins. Avoid excessive consumption of processed foods, sugar, and caffeine.

Skincare Routine: Maintain a consistent skincare routine with gentle cleansers, hydrating moisturizers, and products containing antioxidants and anti-inflammatory ingredients.

Limit Stimulants: Minimize caffeine, nicotine, and alcohol intake, as they can contribute to stress and skin issues.

Seek Support: Talk to friends, family, or a professional counselor to address and manage stress effectively.

Remember that everyone's response to stress is different, and skin reactions can vary. If stress is significantly impacting your skin or overall well-being, consider seeking advice from a dermatologist or healthcare professional. Managing stress not only benefits your skin but also promotes better mental and physical health.

6.2 The Role of Diet and Nutrition

A healthy diet and proper nutrition play a crucial role in promoting radiant and healthy skin. What you eat can affect your skin's appearance, texture, and overall health. Here are some dietary tips and nutrients that are beneficial for your skin:

1. Hydration:

Drink plenty of water throughout the day to keep your skin hydrated and maintain its elasticity.

2. Antioxidants:

Antioxidant-rich foods help protect the skin from free radicals, which can lead to premature aging and skin damage. Include a variety of fruits and vegetables, such as berries, citrus fruits, spinach, kale, and bell peppers.

3. Healthy Fats:

Omega-3 fatty acids found in fatty fish (salmon, mackerel, and sardines), flaxseed, and chia seeds help maintain the skin's moisture barrier and reduce inflammation.

4. Vitamin C:

Vitamin C is essential for collagen production, which keeps the skin firm and youthful. Include foods like citrus fruits, strawberries, kiwi, and broccoli in your diet.

5. Vitamin E:

Vitamin E is another potent antioxidant that protects the skin from damage caused by UV rays and free radicals. Nuts, seeds, avocados, and leafy greens are good sources of vitamin E.

6. Vitamin A and Beta-Carotene:

These nutrients support skin cell turnover and help maintain healthy skin. Consume foods rich in beta-carotene, such as carrots, sweet potatoes, and pumpkin, which are converted to vitamin A in the body.

7. Zinc:

Zinc is involved in skin repair and healing. Foods like oysters, nuts, seeds, and legumes are good sources of zinc.

8. Probiotics:

Probiotics promote a healthy gut, which is linked to better skin health. Yogurt, kefir, sauerkraut, and kimchi are sources of probiotics.

9. Avoid Excessive Sugar and Processed Foods:

High sugar intake can lead to glycation, a process that contributes to skin aging. Minimize consumption of sugary and processed foods.

10. Collagen-Boosting Foods:

Collagen-rich foods like bone broth, fish, chicken, and egg whites can support collagen production in the skin.

11. Limit Alcohol and Caffeine:

Excessive alcohol and caffeine consumption can dehydrate the skin and contribute to inflammation.

12. Maintain a Balanced Diet:

Focus on a well-balanced diet that includes a variety of nutrients to support overall health, which in turn reflects on your skin.

Remember that diet alone cannot solve all skin issues, but it can significantly contribute to healthy, glowing skin. Combine a nutritious diet with a consistent skincare routine and other healthy lifestyle practices, such as regular exercise and stress management, for optimal skin health. If you have specific skin concerns or dietary restrictions, consider consulting with a registered dietitian or dermatologist for personalized advice.

6.3 Beauty Sleep and Skin Repair

Sleep plays a crucial role in the skin's repair and rejuvenation process. During sleep, the body goes through various physiological changes that are essential for skin health and overall well-being. Here's how sleep impacts skin repair:

1. Cellular Repair and Regeneration:

While you sleep, your body's production of growth hormones increases. These hormones are responsible for stimulating cell and tissue repair, including the skin. As a result, the skin's damaged cells are repaired, and new cells are produced.

2. Collagen Production:

Collagen is a protein that provides structural support to the skin, keeping it firm and elastic. During deep sleep, the body produces more collagen, helping to minimize the appearance of wrinkles and fine lines.

3. Blood Flow and Circulation:

During sleep, blood flow to the skin increases. This enhanced circulation ensures that the skin receives essential nutrients and oxygen, promoting skin health and a radiant complexion.

4. Hydration and Moisture Balance:

While sleeping, the body's hydration levels are better balanced, preventing excessive water loss from the skin. This helps maintain the skin's natural moisture and prevents it from becoming dehydrated.

5. Reduction in Inflammation:

Adequate sleep helps reduce inflammation in the body, including the skin. Inflammation can worsen skin conditions like acne, eczema, and psoriasis.

6. Dark Circles and Puffiness:

Sufficient sleep can reduce the appearance of dark circles and under-eye puffiness, as it allows the blood vessels around the eyes to constrict and inflammation to subside.

7. Stress Reduction:

Quality sleep is vital for managing stress, as stress hormones can lead to skin problems like acne breakouts and increased sensitivity.

8. Skin Barrier Function:

Sleep helps maintain the skin's barrier function, preventing irritants and pollutants from penetrating the skin and causing damage.

Tips for Quality Sleep:

Aim for 7-9 hours of sleep per night, as individual needs can vary.

Establish a consistent sleep schedule, going to bed and waking up at the same time each day, even on weekends.

Create a sleep-conducive environment, with a comfortable mattress and pillows, and keep your bedroom cool, dark, and quiet.

Limit exposure to screens (phones, laptops, TVs) before bedtime, as blue light can disrupt sleep.

Engage in relaxing bedtime routines, such as reading, taking a warm bath, or practicing relaxation techniques like meditation.

Prioritizing good-quality sleep not only promotes skin repair but also supports overall health and well-being. If you're experiencing persistent skin issues or sleep disturbances, consider consulting with a dermatologist or healthcare professional for personalized advice and solutions.

Chapter 7: Holistic Approaches to Skincare

7.1 Yoga and Skincare: Finding Balance

Yoga can be a beneficial addition to your skincare routine as it promotes overall well-being, reduces stress, and improves blood circulation, which can lead to healthier and more radiant skin. Here are some yoga practices and poses that can specifically contribute to better skin health:

Pranayama (Breathing Exercises): Deep breathing exercises like Bhramari Pranayama (Humming Bee Breath) and Kapalbhati (Skull-Shining Breath) help oxygenate the blood and improve circulation, nourishing the skin from within.

Surya Namaskar (Sun Salutations): This sequence of yoga poses helps in stretching and toning the entire body, improving blood flow and promoting a healthy glow to the skin.

Twisting Poses: Poses like Ardha Matsyendrasana (Half Lord of the Fishes Pose) and Parivrtta Utkatasana (Revolved Chair Pose) aid in detoxification by massaging the internal organs, which can lead to clearer skin.

Forward Bends: Uttanasana (Standing Forward Bend) and Paschimottanasana (Seated Forward Bend) can calm the mind and reduce stress, which can be beneficial for preventing stress-induced skin issues.

Inversions: Poses like Sirsasana (Headstand) and Sarvangasana (Shoulderstand) increase blood flow to the face, rejuvenating the skin and promoting a youthful appearance.

Matsyasana (Fish Pose): This backbend pose stretches the neck and throat area, helping in reducing thyroid imbalances that could affect the skin.

Balasana (Child's Pose): Relaxing in Child's Pose can help alleviate stress, which is often linked to skin problems like acne and eczema.

Meditation: Incorporating mindfulness and meditation into your yoga practice can reduce stress and promote a sense of calm, which can have a positive impact on skin health.

Facial Yoga: Some yoga practices specifically target facial muscles, which can help reduce tension and wrinkles, promoting a more relaxed and youthful appearance.

Remember that yoga is not a quick fix, and consistent practice is key to experiencing its benefits for overall well-being and skin health. Combined with a balanced diet, proper hydration, and a natural skincare routine, yoga can contribute to healthier and more radiant skin. As always, consult with a healthcare professional or yoga instructor if you have any medical conditions or concerns before starting a new yoga practice.

7.2 Meditation for Skin Health

Meditation can be a powerful tool for improving skin health by reducing stress and promoting overall well-being. Stress is known to have a significant impact on skin health, often exacerbating skin conditions such as acne, eczema, psoriasis, and other inflammatory skin issues. When you meditate regularly, you can experience a range of benefits that positively affect your skin:

Stress Reduction: Meditation helps activate the body's relaxation response, which lowers stress hormones like cortisol. Reduced stress levels can lead to fewer skin flare-ups and a more balanced complexion.

Improved Sleep: Regular meditation can enhance sleep quality, allowing the skin to repair and rejuvenate during the night. Quality sleep is crucial for healthy-looking skin.

Enhanced Blood Circulation: Meditation can improve blood circulation, which delivers essential nutrients and oxygen to the skin cells, promoting a healthy and radiant complexion.

Detoxification: Meditation aids in detoxifying the body by supporting the lymphatic system, which can help eliminate toxins and waste products that may contribute to skin issues.

Emotional Balance: Meditation helps you develop emotional resilience, reducing negative emotional states that can manifest on the skin.

Here's a simple meditation practice you can incorporate into your skincare routine:

Find a Quiet Space: Choose a quiet and comfortable space where you can sit or lie down without distractions.

Focus on Your Breath: Close your eyes and take a few deep breaths. Observe the sensation of your breath as you inhale and exhale. Let go of any tension with each exhale.

Body Scan: Gradually scan your body from head to toe, noticing any areas of tension or discomfort. Allow these areas to relax and release.

Set an Intention: You can set an intention for your meditation, such as "I am taking care of my skin and overall well-being" or "I am letting go of stress and cultivating inner peace."

Focus on the Present: Bring your attention to the present moment. If your mind wanders, gently guide it back to your breath or your chosen point of focus.

Practice Mindfulness: Be aware of any thoughts or emotions that arise during meditation without judgment. Allow them to come and go, returning your focus to the present moment.

End with Gratitude: When you're ready to conclude your meditation, take a few deep breaths, and express gratitude for taking this time for yourself and your skin's well-being.

Remember, consistency is essential in experiencing the benefits of meditation for skin health. Even a few minutes of daily meditation can make a difference. Combined with a holistic approach to skincare, meditation can contribute to a healthier, more radiant complexion.

Skincare is individualized, and what works for one person may not work for another. It's essential to pay attention to your skin's needs and concerns, and if you have specific skin issues, consider consulting with a dermatologist for personalized advice and recommendations.